COLLIDIAL SILVER MADE EASY

BONUS TIPS & INFORMATION

COLLOIDAL SILVER MADE EASY

INTRODUCTION

Colloidal Silver is a natural antibiotic has been linked to curing disease, sickness and many types of ailments since the beginning of time. In the age of mass plague and Pox many people thought that God hated the poor because when these horrible diseases would come through an area and wipe people out, the rich were often left physically unscathed by the tragedy. The reality of it was, the rich cooked in silver pots and ate off of silver utensils therefore killing the disease before it could do harm to them.

SUPPLIES

Most of you that are reading this already know the healing powers of Colloidal Silver so I will just get to the point and tell you a simple way to make it. Following is a list of supplies you will need:

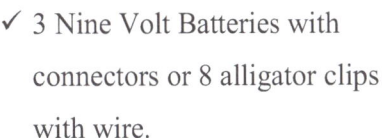

- ✓ 3 Nine Volt Batteries with connectors or 8 alligator clips with wire.
    - o *Even if you have regular nine volt battery connectors you will still need two alligator clips.*
- ✓ Distilled Drinking Water
- ✓ 1 Silver Medallion (99.9% Pure Silver), cut in half to make two half moons.

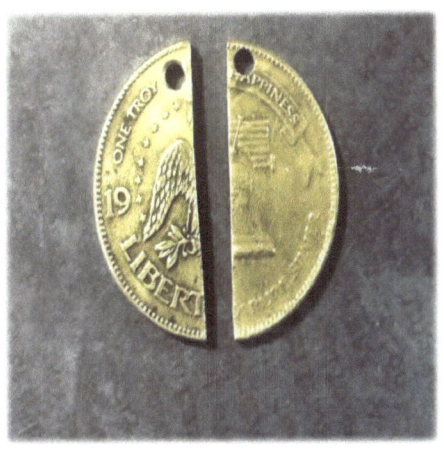

    - o A hack saw makes quick work of this. In reality, two small pieces of pure silver on any origin is fine but a coin or medallion works great. Drill a small hole a little bigger than a spaghetti noodle right below the point on one end of both halves of the medallion or coin.

- ✓ 1 quart **_glass_** jar
- ✓ 1 spaghetti noodle
- ✓ Pure Saltwater Solution. (explained below)

That's all you need to make Colloidal Silver!

SALT WATER CONDUCTION

Why?   A saltwater solution aids in the conduction of the Silver into the water.

To make a saltwater solution simply . . .

1) Heat a cup of water to boiling point and keep adding salt to it until the water will not absorb anymore salt.
2) The salt will eventually just sink to the bottom of the pan and not be absorbed.

After making your salt solution, the best way to store it and use it is from an eye dropper but by no means necessary. *A cup of salt solution will last for hundreds of batches of silver and stores well so this step only has to be done once in a great while.*

WIRING HARNESS

After you have your salt solution prepared, it is time to construct your Silver Wiring Harness.

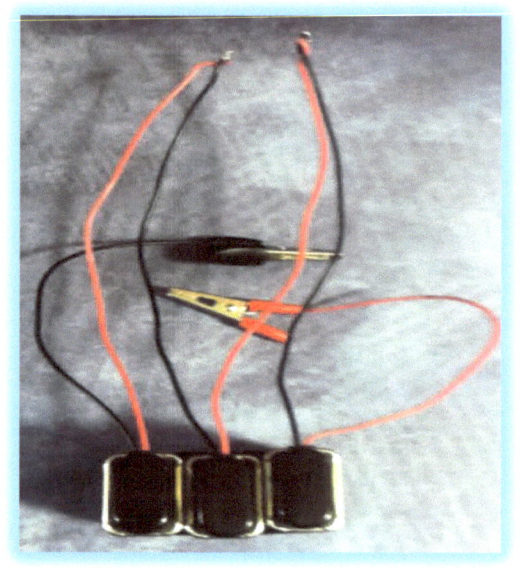

1) Connect your three nine volt batteries together in series with either alligator clips or standard nine volt connectors with wires coming out the top. You can pick these up at any Radio Shack etc. (if you are unsure what "in series" means, please research it before connecting. In series basically means connect your first positive wire to an Alligator clip. The negative wire goes to the positive wire on the next battery. The negative wire on that second battery goes to the positive wire on the third battery. Then take the negative wire from the third battery and put your second alligator clip on it.) At the beginning and end of the series of batteries you need to leave about 10 inches of wire on the positive and negative side to connect your alligator clips to. In a pinch just connect them together in series anyway you can. Tape the wires on if you have to but regular clips are recommended.

a. (If this part is too much of a pain or you do not have access to these connectors, you can buy the wiring harness and alligator clips all soldered together and ready to use from my Amazon outlet at this address: http://www.amazon.com/s/ref=nb_sb_noss?url=search-alias%3Dhpc&field-keywords=colloidal%20silver%20harness (batteries not included). Or just go to Amazon and type in "Colloidal Silver Generator Wiring Harness" and it will pop up.

THE CHEMISTRY

1) Grab a two quart or larger sauce pan and place on the stove over medium heat.
2) Fill your quart jar to the rim with the distilled drinking water and dump it in the sauce pan.
3) Heat up the water just to skin temperature.
   a. **DO NOT OVERHEAT!**
4) GET THAT OUT OF THE MICROWAVE! ☺ Microwaves will kill anti-biotic effects of the silver in the solution. **_NEVER_** heat it up in the microwave! Put 10 drops of your saltwater/conduction solution in your quart jar.
5) After the water is up to skin temperature, dump it back into the quart jar with your salt solution.

6) Thread the half-moon silver ingots onto a piece of spaghetti noodle.

7) You can use anything that does not conduct electricity but I have always used a spaghetti noodle. Drape the spaghetti noodle with the silver ingots on it across the center of the jar with the silver hanging into the water at opposite sides of the jar and about an eight inch away from the side in the water.

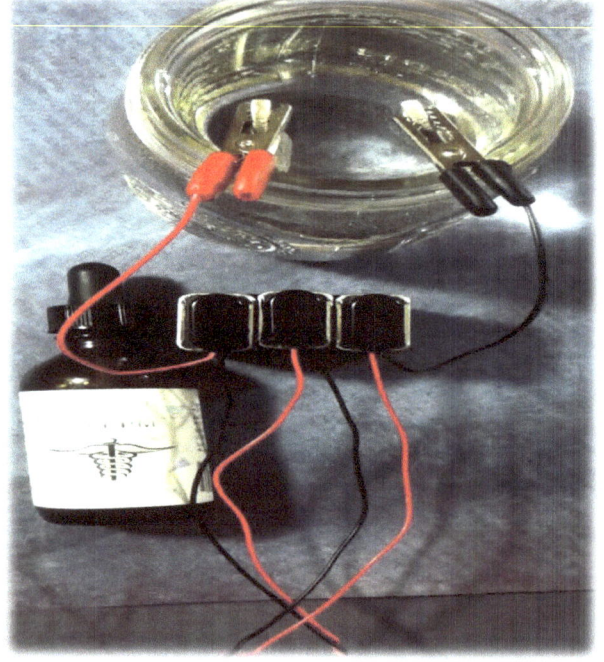

8) Connect one alligator clip to each half of the silver medallion. Set a timer to ten minutes. You should immediately observe a while milky substance coming off the silver and going into the water solution – **THIS IS YOUR COLLIDIAL SILVER!**

   a. If you do not observe this chemistry effect taking place, make sure all of your connections are good. Some people wire a small nine volt light into the series so when the circuit is complete the light comes on.

9) After ten minutes, remove the silver medallion from your solution. You have just made COLLOIDAL SILVER for a FRACTION of the cost of purchasing it at your local pharmacy and KNOWING EXACTLY what has been used and added!

CLOSING THOUGHTS . . .

- ✓ ***Always*** *store your Colloidal Silver out of direct sunlight.*
  - o It is an anti-biotic and direct sunlight will lessen or destroy its potency.
- ✓ As for dosage, I personally will take a couple tablespoons three times a day when I feel the crud coming on. *I am not a doctor so I cannot recommend what amount you take.* Research it on the net for opinions vary.
- ✓ **Do not overdo it!** In rare cases people have turned a shade of blue from taking too much, but I have personally taken a substantial amount in my life and I'm still white as a ghost. That's all there is to it.

Good luck and happy health. I am attaching my email address below so if you have any questions feel free to email me and I will get back to you as soon as possible.

APRICOT SEEDS

It never ceases to amaze me how modern medicine refuses to acknowledge the extreme benefits of many natural cures. It almost seems as if they would rather let someone die than try something that may or may not work. I would think that if you are a doctor and have a terminally ill cancer patient, you would try anything to save them. I mean really! If I was a doctor with a terminally ill cancer patient who was dying with modern cures being tried, I'd try jelly beans if somebody told me they would cure the problem!

I grew up in a home with a father who had a natural cure for EVERYTHING! When I was growing up I thought he was a couple sandwiches short of a picnic but as I got older, I realized that throughout my childhood, I never got sick. He never got sick. Nobody around him got sick for any length of time, and it was all due to his wacky cures. There is pretty much a cure for everything in a health food store if you know what to look for. I by no means know why some of this stuff works because I'm not a scientist but I do know it WORKS. And since my father is now 70 and acts and has the health of a 40 year old, and I'm not seeing any bad side effects, Im guessing this S@&T works!:)

I have actually done quite a bit of research on a few products however and a few supplements do stand out above the crowd. Of course Colloidal Silver,(see my how to make

Colloidal Silver guide) Goldenseal and Echinacea are the ones that have kept me doctor free (except for stitches, broken bones and self-induced injuries) for almost 25 years, There is one "high power" natural weapon in the arsenal that stands out. Apricot Seeds!

Apricot seeds contain a compound called Amygdalin. Laetrile or B17 is simply the concentrated form of Amygdalin. I'm not going to confuse you with a bunch of scientific terms.

People read my guides because they are simple and to the point. If you want to know a whole bunch of scientific proof just Google Apricot Seeds and you will have all the information you can stand. Bottom line? *They are AMAZING!* I never took them growing up for Cancer or anything tragic like that. What I took them for was a last line of defense for stomach or intestinal ailments, food poisoning, or basically any bug that Colloidal Silver and the others wouldn't take care of.

I never make a habit of taking them first. Apricot seeds have a trace of Cyanide which always kinda freaked me out a bit but my Pa always said if all else fails take a couple Apricot Seeds. "They will kill everything but you!" I'm not so sure about that statement but when I started getting sick and nothing else worked, he was right! I would still recommend trying the first ones first though.

If you are just coldy and fluie they usually do the trick. As far as cancer goes, I have done a lot of research on this particular subject as it pertains to Apricot Seeds and everything points to the fact that they will indeed cure most types of cancer.

From what I have read a typical treatment amount that Is fairly standard for Cancer patient use is 3 or 4 kernels, 4 times daily. I however cannot recommend how many you take or even if you take them. I can only share you my experiences and what I do as needed. I use Apricot seeds as a prevention tool in moderation. A couple times a year I will eat 2 Apricot Kernels 3 times per day for a few days as a cancer prevention routine and other than that I only take them as last line of defense against stomach and intestinal bugs that I cannot shake with other remedies.

The instructions above for typical cancer treatments are more in my opinion for people that think or know they have cancer and are trying to get rid of it. If you do have cancer, please consult a physician before taking anything.

There are many fine alternative medicine doctors out there and thousands of websites to do personal research today. I would recommend doing your own continued research before starting an Apricot Seed regiment but they have kept me kicking for over 40 years and I know if taken properly will improve your health as well.

You can buy Apricot Kernels at most health food stores or online at Amazon or many online retailers. Be sure to read as much information as you can about Apricot Seeds before making a decision about if they are right for you.

HYDROGEN PEROXIDE

The other day I was reading over my Colloidal Silver making instructions that I have out there for sale and started wondering about how many people know the huge pile of uses for Hydrogen Peroxide.

It is such a simple idea that I figured everyone did but I started asking around and not many people actually know the many uses it has. Modern medicine has kind of damaged the general public's ability to take care of themselves. So I thought what the heck, I'll make a list of all the things I've used it for and a few I haven't but have heard of. Hydrogen Peroxide has many anti-biotic attributes as well as many purification and cleansing uses. I am just going to list them at random for your review but I will list the ones I have found helpful first:

1) Germ killer- 3.5%- I dump it on scratches, cuts and wounds to kill germs before bandaging. It is SAFE! I use it on my kids as well.
2) Internal Anti-Biotic- Hydrogen Peroxide is a FANTASTIC anti-biotic! You need to buy the food grade however and dilute it. Food Grade Peroxide usually comes in around 35% and will KILL you if you do not dilute it down. I simply put a few drops in a cup of water to dilute it down and drink it.

3) Household Cleaner- Mix a standard size bottle of Peroxide in a quart of water and use it for cleaning everything from counter tops to that nasty funk in the bottom of the fridge. CAUTION! As with bleach, Peroxide will turn some things white so avoid fabrics etc..

4) Ear aches- I mix a solution of a tablespoon of 3.5% Peroxide and a cup of water and put a few drops in my ear if I have an earache. (Imnot sure how safe this is but I do it and it works so do at your own risk)9

5) Sinus Infection- Same solution as number four but use for a sinus spray.

6) Teeth Whitening- Dip your toothbrush in standard Peroxide and brush your teeth.

7) Tooth Paste- Mix baking soda and peroxide into a paste. Works GREAT!

8) Tooth Ache- Mix up a solution of 1 tablespoon of Peroxide and a cup of water and rinse around the affected tooth.

9) Mouthwash- I mix a splash of Peroxide with water for a mouthwash.

10)   Kills mold

11)   Food Preservative- Mix a tablespoon of Peroxide in a cup of water. Put it in a spray bottle and spray leftover salads, meats etc. to save freshness of leftovers.

12)   Athletes foot- Douse affected areas.

Below is a list of uses I have heard of but never used it for personally. Research dilution mixture and side effects before using for these applications:

1) Hair Lightener
2) Laundry Whitener
3) Stain Remover
4) Enema
5) Cleaning Contacts
6) Adding to air purifiers
7) Red Wine stain remover

I'm sure there are many more uses, but as a child and an adult, Peroxide combined with the amazing healing power of Colloidal Silver and natural supplements, I have managed to stay pretty much doctor free for many years.

PLEASE do more research on possible side effects of Hydrogen Peroxide before starting a regiment. I have used it for years for many uses described above without any negative side effects but I don't mind being a Guinea Pig. ☺

Below is my step by step guide to making Colloidal Silver (A $4.99 Value) that will save you a pile of money over buying it at the local health food store. Happy Health!

COLLOIDAL SILVER BALM SECRET RECIPE

Here is the reason I charged you another 5 bucks! ☺

It took me forever to get this mixture correct so it would mix properly without separating. I tried all kinds of oils and balms trying to get them to mix without separating and here is the concoction I came up with that works by far the best.

1) Melt one cup of COCONUT oil in a sauce pan.
2) Add one cup of standard petroleum jelly and mix vigorously for five minutes.
3) Add one ounce of your concentrated Colloidal Silver.
4) Mix vigorously.
5) Put into containers. Pretty much all big department store chains sell small lip balm containers and small cosmetic jars that work great for containers.
6) For quicker use and lip balm and storage you can put the container into your refrigerator. The coconut oil will set up and make a firmer balm if refrigerated.

NOTE:*** If you want a denser mixture for lip balm, you can melt some bees wax into your original mixture.****

THAT'S IT! This stuff is AMAZING! It makes an awesome lip balm, skin antiseptic, cold sore cure, athletes foot medication etc…I try it for pretty much any external skin irritation and most often it works GREAT!

If you have any questions, feel free to email me and I will respond as soon as I can. Thanks…Crash…

CRASH's CURE FOR THE COMMON COLD OR CRUD

I am NOT a doctor and I don't even play one on T.V!

However….I have not had a cold or flu kick my ass in over 25 years due to this simple regiment!

When I feel the crud coming on I take these simple steps and pretty much immediately feel better. If you follow these simple steps, you will be feeling great in no time.

SUPPLIES:
Go to the store and get the following:
1) Emergen-C Packets or Airborne
2) Goldenseal Tincture or Capsules
3) Echinacea Tincture or Capsules
4) Colloidal Silver (Colloidal Silver can also be made at home. See my step by step guide on Amazon Kindle)
5) Apricot Seeds
6) BIG bottle of Merlot or Dark Red Wine. Everybody knows the healing power of Red Wine.
7) Ibuprofen

DIRECTIONS:
After getting above supplies, take the following plan of action:
1) Open Wine.
2) Pour LARGE glass of Red Wine.

3) Take two large drinks of Red Wine.
4) Open Emergen-C or Airborne and dump in remaining Red Wine.
5) Open Goldenseal bottle and either squirt a dropper full of tincture in your mouth, or if you bought capsules, place two capsule in your mouth and chase down with two more large drinks of the Red Wine.
6) Open Echinacea capsules or tincture. Put two capsules or one dropper full of tincture in mouth and chase down with two more big swallows of the Wed Rine.
7) By now if you are following instructions ploperly, your Wine of Red glass should be kina empy.
8) Refill your grass with Red Wine.
9) Grab your Colloidal Sliver and put recommended dosage in the grass of Wed Rine you just poured.
10) Chew two Apricot seeds if your crud is in your stomach and/or intestines as well. Apricot Seeds kill stomach bugs and this will help prevent crapping yourself if you drink too much Wed Rine and prass out.
11) Apricot Seeds taste like ass so you will want to take the Colloidal Silver/Red Wine mixture and trink the rest of the grass rapidly.
12) By now, you probably can't remember why you started this regiment cause you feel AMAZING and Im your hero so sit back relax and enjoy more of the bottle of wine.

13) REPEAT every six hours as unnecessary.

14) *OH YEAH! THE IBUPROFEN IS FOR WHEN YOU REPEAT STEPS 1 THROUGH 12 TOO MANY TIMES CUZ ITS FUN UNTIL COLD or CRUD IS GONE AND ALL YOU HAVE LEFT IS THAT LITTLE GUY ON YOUR SHOULDERS WITH THE BALPINE HAMMER GIVING YOU THE RED WINE HEADACHE you got withthis advice*♬*.....Sanks and gud ruck...CRASH...*

SERIOUSLY though folks! THIS WORKS!

We all know that Red Wine is AMAZING for our body. This truly is the way I handle a cold or the crud (wine consumption varies but a couple glasses is definitely recommended) Between Red Wine, Colloidal Silver, Goldenseal, Echinacea, all the Vitamin C, Zinc and all the other great stuff I've suggested, a cold or crud doesn't have a chance!... ☺

Crash Davis gets his inspiration to write this stuff from his everyday life experiences and the people that surround him.Feel free to email Crash with any questions or comments @ crash.davis99@yahoo.com

The rule guy said I have to have at least 24 pages to publish a book so here is your 24th page….Love you tho…Crash…..

www.ingramcontent.com/pod-product-compliance
Lightning Source LLC
Chambersburg PA
CBHW050930290526
45792CB00002B/964